I0842099

Table of Contents

Introduction

Some people feel like they've been dieting forever, have experimented with all sorts of regimens, and yet they are always hungry and never in the shape they'd like to be.

At the same time, there are individuals who can eat whatever they feel like and yet they don't gain any weight. They've never been on a diet or done anything to regulate their weight, but any amount of calories they consume is immediately burned instead of stored.

What's the reason for that? Their metabolism.

People with a fast metabolism don't have problems maintaining their weight as their system breaks down food pretty quickly. While that might be in their genes or thanks to the muscles they've built through exercising for years, there are ways you can speed up your metabolism and be like them.

The most effective way to improve your metabolism is by fixing your diet and in this guide for beginners, you'll learn how.

Before that, however, you need to understand how your metabolism works and why it's so important. Then, you'll also find out ways to control it. By increasing your metabolic rate with the right foods and diet plan, you can be in shape before you know it and in the most natural way.

If done right, you can have a fast metabolism even when you get back to eating normally. There are additional benefits, though, related to the other functions of the metabolism. Digestion is only one of them. It's also responsible for blood circulation, clearing toxins out of the body and regulating body heat.

That means once you increase your metabolism thanks to the right diet, you will improve your overall well-being by cleansing your system, strengthening the immune system, having better skin, boosted mood, and more.

Assuming you're only doing this to lose weight, you should expect rapid weight loss. As a result of quickly digesting any calories you consume and burning fat, you will be able to look your best.

To truly grasp the role of metabolism, you should understand how it works. That will be covered in the next chapter of the book. You'll learn its main phases, the metabolic processes it's responsible for and how each creates balance in our body. After that, we'll talk about metabolic disorder as you might be having one of the symptoms of such a dysfunction without realizing it. If you do, you'll learn new ways to treat it.

Later in the book, you will understand how to calculate your ideal body weight. Setting it as a goal will help you have a direction and track your progress. Also, it's key to aim at that body weight and nothing less if you want to stay healthy, positive and with a clear mind.

You'll also find a list of metabolism-boosting foods. Even before you check out the diet plan we've prepared for you, you can start making small changes to your daily menu by removing the foods that slow your metabolism and replacing them with those that speed it up. You might want to keep eating this way even when you get to your ideal weight.

Your metabolism is more important than you give it credit for.

Before we begin exploring its functions and how to make it faster, let's see what makes it vital for our organism.

It's wrongly assumed that our metabolism is the rate with which calories are burnt. It's about more than that and the key word here is 'energy'.

Our metabolism is a set of functions related to how our cells are given energy and how they use it. Thanks to these processes, not just humans but all living organisms can exist, move, grow and reproduce. It's because of that energy extracted from food that we are capable of living and thriving.

A well-sustained metabolism helps all vital functions from cellular repair to our ability to think and perform during the day. Any imbalance in it affects our health negatively and weakens our immune system, which in turn leads to diseases.

Look at this guide not just as the solution to your weight problems, but a way to take better care of your body by restarting your metabolism and thus becoming healthier and happier.

You might even find out that many physical, mental or spiritual issues you've been struggling with will finally disappear once and for all. That's because you might have been consuming too much food too often, which prevents the body from digesting it properly and turning it into the energy that it uses to build and repair cells.

Speeding up your metabolism will help you reach out the ideal weight and find fulfillment and clarity. You will basically teach your organism how to extract energy from the right foods at the right speed and use these nutrients to help all other functions in the system.

Let's begin your journey to understanding how the metabolism works exactly so you can kickstart it.

How Does The Metabolism Work?

A metabolism is a set of chemical processes occurring in living cells. It's also the combination of changes happening in the body after absorbing the nutrients of food and turning them into energy that allows our cells to grow and reproduce.

Phases

Metabolism can be broken down into 2 main phases that are interdependent - anabolism and catabolism. These are basically the processes of building molecules and breaking them down.

One of the biggest misconceptions about the metabolism is to mistake it for either anabolism or catabolism. These 2 are completely different processes and only as a result of both of these functions do we provide our body with the energy it needs to grow and survive.

They also create a metabolic cycle - the creation of molecules as a result of anabolism, which are then broken down by the catabolic process. Let's talk about each phase separately.

Anabolism requires energy to organize simple compounds in the body and build the molecules we need. The anabolic hormones include testosterone, estrogen, insulin and the growth hormone.

Catabolism, on the other hand, is the release of energy after breaking down complex molecules into smaller ones. Examples of this process are when protein is broken down and turned into amino acids or glucose, and also fat burn.

Metabolic functions

Here are the main functions of our metabolism and how each contributes to not just maintaining our weight but also being in good health.

Energy production. - We need energy to live well and do all the things we fill our precious time with during the day. That energy comes from not just consuming food but converting the fuel from it and turning it into energy. The metabolism does all this and thus gives us the power to move, think, survive and grow.

It keeps us alive. - Keep in mind that our metabolism is working at any moment of our life. It starts the second we are born and death comes when it stops functioning. Until then, all the chemical processes in our body are responsible for allowing us to use the energy extracted from food to exist and thrive. That energy is used not just when we're moving. Plenty of other functions are going on even when we are still, such as breathing, repairing cells and growing new ones, the circulation of the blood, the balancing of hormone levels, and more.

Cell growth. - The metabolism is literally inside every cell of the body. Each cell itself converts the new energy released after the digestion of foods into smaller molecules. They are even richer in energy and are then used to produce new cells and help the development of existing ones.

Cell division and repair. - Cell division, or mitosis, is a vital process for a number of reasons. For a start, it is the reason why we become adults - by increasing the size of our organisms. Second, it's related to reproduction as it plays a big part in forming sperm and eggs. Third, it repairs tissue and injuries such as a cut to the skin. With this last function, the metabolism can heal damaged cells.

Breaking down fat. - Your metabolism is responsible for fat breakdown. This metabolized fat is then stored for later, in case the body needs energy to function but isn't receiving it from food for a long time, such as during sleep, when on a diet, or else. And this is why weight management has a lot to do with what your metabolic rate is like. While a slow metabolism won't burn all the fat or enough of it until it's time for the next meal, a fast one will break it down and prevent you from gaining any excess weight.

Extracting the nutrients from food. - Digestion isn't just about melting fat. Before that, your metabolism makes sure you get the most out of the food you eat on a daily basis by absorbing its nutrients such as vitamins, minerals, proteins, fats, carbs, and water.

Looking younger. - Cell renewal happens in the skin too. With a well-functioning metabolism, that process will be ongoing and can even slow down aging. If your skin repairs and its cells renew themselves, it can also exfoliate itself, make you look energized and stay smooth. Additionally, with a good diet you can control how it reverses the damage of aging, such as sunburn or the negative effects of other environmental factors.

Achieving your health and fitness goals. - Last but not least, your metabolism can be a stepping stone to accomplishing your life goals, feeling good in your skin and being happy and fulfilled. Because health comes first and we can manage it by recharging our metabolism, it can also be the foundation of what we eat and how active we are. Which, in turn, cures depression, heals anxiety, makes us productive, positive and successful.

To summarize, your metabolism is the reason you are alive, breathing and thinking, and repairing any damage on your body. It's worth taking good care of it and knowing more about the chemical processes in our organism so we can make the most of its functions. To continue with the basics of how the metabolism works, let's see what defines your metabolic rate.

Factors your basal metabolic rate depends on

The basal metabolic rate, or BMR, is the number of calories the body is burning when resting. Or in other words, the energy expenditure for a certain period of time. This rate is linked to your tendency to lose or gain weight.

Two people consuming the same amount of calories in a day, but with a different BMR, will have completely different body structures. The one with a low basal metabolic rate will burn less fat even if they are as active during the day as the person with a higher BMR.

Let's see what factors have a say in this. While not all of them are under your control, you'll notice plenty that you can take action upon and thus increase the rate with which your metabolism uses energy at rest.

Genetic factors

Body size. - A larger body would have a higher metabolic rate. That includes an obese person as well as a tall one. In most cases, it's genetics and there's nothing you can do about it. But that's just one part of the equation. Let's see what else your energy expenditure rate consists of.

Body weight composition. - A much more important factor than the size of your body is what this weight is composed of. Back to the example of a tall person. He has a metabolic advantage and can eat more while burning it all and not gaining weight. That's because the surface of his body is more, which requires more energy to sustain it (even at rest) as opposed to a short person.

Age. - It's a well-known fact that kids need more energy as there's a lot more going on in their body. Infants and teenagers are experiencing something called rapid growth up until they enter adulthood, after which that process slows down. The more we age, the slower our metabolism gets.

Gender. - Men have a bit of an advantage here due to the less amount of fat and the more muscles they have compared to women. Although, of course, females who take good care of their bodies throughout their life by maintaining a healthy diet and exercising, won't have a low metabolic rate because of their gender.

Environmental factors

Climate. - If you're living in a more tropical place, your body will use more of its energy to keep you cool. Even better for your metabolic rate if that continues for the whole year and you don't have winter there. But the same goes for people living in colder countries. In their case, the metabolism would be a bit faster than those living in areas with average climate as it will want to keep the body warm enough.

Hormonal imbalance. - Any imbalance in your hormone levels leads to either gaining or losing weight, fatigue, sweating, irregular heartbeat, losing bone mass, and more. Each of these affects how your metabolism is working too. While it could be genetic, it's part of the Environmental factors section of this book because you hormonal imbalance can be managed and even treated. Also, that might not be running in your family, but be a result of life stages such as puberty or menopause. It could also be permanent or a consequence of stress and anxiety, a bad diet, sleep deprivation, and more.

Medications. - Another outer factor that can cause variation in the basal metabolic rate is any medication you might be taking and, in particular, its side effects. That could be antidepressants or a more serious drug that's prescribed to you by a specialist, but which leads to weight gain, fatigue or else, that then decrease your metabolic rate.

Lifestyle factors

Physical activity. - Any form of exercise burns energy so the organism uses up glucose which then needs to be restored. The more often you work out, the more you increase your metabolic rate even when resting.

Diet. - The next key item on the list is food. What you eat shapes your metabolism and how fast it functions. While some people limit their calorie intake in order to lose weight, they actually lower their metabolic rate. The body is under pressure and adapts to that stressful situation by using less energy to absorb the smaller amount of calories you're now consuming. The longer you're following a low-carb or low-fat diet, the more muscle tissue you lose, which is also affecting your metabolism negatively. At this point, and especially after 30-60 days of such dieting, your body needs much less fuel than usual and has less muscle that requires energy to exist. So your metabolism is now slower than ever. That's also what experts call a plateau. It's when a diet plan is no longer effective and the individual should go back to eating more calories per day, or make other changes in their lifestyle such as adding regular exercise, to reach the average metabolic rate again.

Body temperature. - Similar to living in a cold or warm area, you can make the body use more energy to keep you cooler or warmer at certain times of the day. That can happen by sleeping in a cool room and spending enough time outside during the winter. Or exercising when it's hot, for example, to double the effect of increasing your body temperature and needing energy to stay cool.

Stress levels. - Whenever you're stressed out, you activate the body's fight or flight response. That means the levels of the stress hormone cortisol spike and you enter survival mode. Then, your insulin levels increase and another one of the main stress hormones, norepinephrine, depletes and that slows down the metabolic response. That's why whenever you read a guide on anything health-related, especially when talking about speeding up your metabolism, there will always be tips on how to reduce stress too. That's closely related to whether or not your organism functions well and you have a healthy body and mind. We'll talk more about this in the next section of the guide where you'll learn some simple ways to remove stress from your life and thus fix your metabolism.

Muscle mass. - One of the many benefits of regular physical activity is gaining more muscle mass. However, this requires more energy than fat. Which means the more muscles you have, the more calories you'll be burning even if you don't move much.

Sleep. - Getting a good night's sleep is one of the many ways to keep your metabolism strong and healthy. However, when you're having trouble falling asleep, wake up at night due to snoring, stress or bad sleeping habits and then can't go back to sleep, you end up being sleep deprived. This has many metabolic consequences such as not being able to control your appetite, gaining weight, hormonal imbalance, preventing the body from metabolizing all the nutrients from foods, increasing the insulin and cortisol levels, and much more. It's proven that even one night with poor sleep can have serious consequences on your metabolism.

Health issues. - If you've been injured, have found a disease that can be cured, or just caught the flu, your metabolic rate might double as it has more tissue to repair.

Everybody's metabolism is different and variations in the basal metabolic rate occur due to any change in the lifestyle of the individual. So for a start, make a list of the factors above and personalize it. See how each of the things influencing the speed with which you burn energy is contributing to your fat loss and good health. Then, define the influences that have the opposite effect and encourage weight gain. These are the factors you should take into consideration, so make a plan on how to remove them.

For example, if your physical activity is one weak point of yours, you can join a gym and start lifting weights 3 times a week. After a month, you can add 2 cardio sessions per week too. Having 5 workouts on a weekly basis is a great way to speed up your metabolism by not just burning more fat but also building muscle. This means you'll be activating both the anabolic and catabolic processes with the 2 types of exercises. Each contributes to how your body functions in a different way. The 2 phases complement each other and, in turn, give you a toned body with less fat.

But that's just one example. The point is to know what causes your metabolism to be slower than its average speed and do something about it. Let's find out how to do that naturally:

How to Naturally Increase Your Metabolic Rate

To make it easier for you, I'll follow the order of the items presented above. Now that you know what causes a lower metabolic rate and have identified your weaknesses, here are some ideas on what to do about almost all of the negative influences you just read about:

Change your body composition.

It's not the end of the world if your metabolic rate is lower due to things such as entering your 40s, being shorter, or female. There are plenty of other habits you can build that will affect positively the rest of the factors influencing the speed of your metabolism. For a start, that's your body composition. And it's a result of the food you consume and the energy your body uses to digest it. These can be under your control with the right diet and regular exercise. Additionally, when turning that into your lifestyle, you'll build muscle and thus speed up your metabolism. Also, you'll lose fat and that itself will increase your metabolic rate.

Many people give up and don't even try because they've always been obese. That could be due to always being on a diet and never giving your body a chance to actually stop storing fat and burn all that you eat naturally. It might be time to try this. It's the natural way to get in shape and will have long-term positive effects on your metabolism.

Sleep in a cooler room.

Sleep experts suggest we keep our bedrooms cool. One of the many benefits of that is keeping our bodies cool at night promotes the process of burning energy at all times.

Our body temperature naturally decreases when we get to sleep. To make the most of this, help your body stay this way by sleeping in a cool room. In addition, such an environment is great for your sleep cycle. A warm sleeping environment, on the other hand, disturbs your deep sleep stage and might even wake you up.

Fix your hormones.

A good first step that concerns every aspect of your health is to get your hormones tested and see if there are any specific inconsistencies. That will help you find out (and get some guidelines from a specialist) what exactly you can do to balance a certain hormone.

But there are plenty of tips to follow that will affect your hormone levels in general. They are proven, natural and even fun to do. In fact, taking these steps and turning them into a habit can increase your lifespans and lead to having a happy and fulfilled life over the next decades.

Here are some ways to treat hormonal imbalance that will also improve your metabolism:

Eat plenty of protein - you might even want to include it in every meal;
Ditch sugar-sweetened drinks;
Add fiber to your diet;
Stop overeating;
Eat the good fats, not chemically altered fats such as cooking oil or margarine;
Look where chemicals might be hidden in your home (that could be your mattress, cleaners, beauty products, and plastics);
Clean your home better to get rid of them;
Add plants to your home to have clean and fresh air indoors;
Be careful with any medicine or even supplement you're taking as each might change your hormones;
Reach hormone balance with herbs;
Reset your leptin sensitivity;

Take care of your emotional health;
Use essential oils;
Don't take birth control;
Sop eating foods that cause inflammation such as sugar, dairy and processed meat;
Get enough omega 3 per day.

Start exercising on a regular basis.

One of the most common tips you'll hear if you ask people how to make your metabolism work faster is to begin exercising. But it's not just that. Thanks to some kind of physical activity during the day, you can rev your metabolism all day long. That means it's always going to be absorbing nutrients from food and turning them into energy faster even when you're resting.

To take this further, you should move your workout to the morning. Kickstarting your day and metabolism by exercising when you get up is a practical way to be burning calories till the evening.

Do both cardio and weight lifting.

Once you make working out regularly a habit, you can make changes to get better results. That doesn't mean you need to sweat for more than 45-60 minutes a day. It just means you should activate both the anabolic and catabolic processes. Which means doing not just cardio or lifting only weights, but both of these.

Or you could do strength training 3 times a week and make time for metabolic conditioning, or cardio, twice a week.

Over time, you'll find what works best for you. You might notice cardio in the early morning makes you tired for the rest of the day, in which case it's better to do it later in the day. As for weight training, maybe you enjoy it so much that you can do it more times a week. It's okay to focus on one of these 2 types of exercises more. Building more muscles will become your new thing and that will fix your metabolism in no time.

Identify your biggest stressors.

Moving onto the mental health aspect of increasing your metabolic rate. It all begins by awareness. There could be many things in your surroundings or in your mind that are making your anxious. They aren't always obvious until you dig deeper. So have an honest conversation with yourself and see what you're worried about, what you fear or the external factors in your life that bring pressure. Once you define these stressors, you can do something about each.

Some people are stressed out so often that it becomes their normal state and eventually turns into chronic stress syndrome. Before you get there, you should take back control of your peace of mind. Do that by eliminating anything that's stressing you too much. That could be toxic people in your circle who are too negative or judgmental. It could also be a toxic relationship that you're holding onto but which doesn't have any future. It's best to let it go even if it hurts now. It's good for both people involved in it.

Some stressors are related to your work life. It could be bad time management if you're always in a hurry, a job you don't like that makes you miserable, a new client that gives you many deadlines and you just can't seem to keep up. Whatever the case, that's overwhelming and making you miserable. As a result, your health suffers.

Some ways to fight stress include:

Surround yourself with happy people;
Listening to music;
Being in nature more often;
Having some 'me' time daily;
Breathing techniques;
Lighting a candle;
Chewing gum;
Cuddling;
Laughing;
Dancing;
Taking a break from work;
And more.

Have a relaxing evening routine.

Another great way to reduce your stress levels is to dedicate your time before bed to relaxing activities and nothing too stressful. If you do that, you will go to bed with an empty mind, will sleep well and wake up fresh and ready to get some work done. If you don't do that, however, you'll take your problems with you in bed and will ruin your rest.

A good evening routine won't include any food or beverages, especially not alcohol or caffeine. Have a snack an hour before that and leave the next one for tomorrow morning when you can have a nutritious breakfast.

Ditch technology too as the blue light it emits disturbs your sleep and keeps your brain active. Social media is pretty bad for your mental health. So during this relaxing period, forget about it. It's best to keep your phone away from your bed too.

The things you can do instead include reading and writing, talking to a loved one, stretching, doing yoga or meditating, decluttering at home, preparing for tomorrow.

Take breaks during the day.

People underestimate the power of frequent breaks. But they are necessary not just to boost our productivity during the workday, but so we can recharge our brain and keep it healthy.

Napping during the day is one way to do that. It's also good for your stress levels to work on a task for around 45 minutes after which you should go do something else for 5-15 minutes. It's refreshing and actually leads to getting more done.

Also, employees who take vacations more often are happier and healthier.

Fix your sleeping schedule.

Getting better sleep begins by waking up and going to bed at the same time every day. Sticking to a routine is good for your sleep-wake cycle and for getting a solid sleep every night. Your metabolism will be happy about this too.

Start eating metabolism-boosting foods.

Fixing your diet is another crucial element and you'll see a whole chapter later in this guide dedicated to the right foods you should eat. What's more, you'll find out what not to eat and what small changes you can make to your eating habits and routines for better digestion.

Now you know how your metabolism works, why it matters so much, what determined whether or not your basal metabolic rate will be high enough to help you burn more calories, and how to fix some of the weak points in your environment and lifestyle so you can improve your metabolism.

All that information will be useful whenever you decide to go on a diet. It's also the foundation of your workouts as you now know what 2 processes are being activated whenever you do certain types of exercises. Additionally, any little things you do during the day and habit you've formed over the years somehow affects your metabolism. Information is powerful, tough, and now you can use it to your advantage.

Set some time aside to understand what you might be doing wrong that's resulting in a low metabolic rate. The secret to weight management is hidden there too. But of course, it all comes down to your diet. We'll talk about this in details later on. Now, let's move onto discussing why the metabolic processes fail sometimes, which leads to metabolic dysfunctions, and how to treat that.

Metabolic Dysfunction

A metabolic dysfunction, or metabolic disorder, is any abnormality in the metabolic process. It's when certain chemical reactions in the body cause metabolism problems. The disorder is most often inherited and means there are too many or not enough substances in the system that are necessary for the metabolism to work properly at all times.

There are many forms, causes and treatments for the different metabolic disorders. We'll now go through the symptoms so you can find out whether you have such a dysfunction, after which we'll discuss solutions.

Symptoms

The symptoms below may occur slowly over the ages but also suddenly. The speed of their progress can vary too.

In the case of an inherited metabolic disorder, you might notice some of the following:

Losing weight;
Lack of appetite;
Fatigue;
Skin pigmentation;
Slow development;
Seizures;
Coma.

The above can be experienced in most other types of metabolic dysfunction too. But here are some more symptoms you might notice depending on the cause of the condition. As you might see, some are more severe than others:

Liver failure;
Weaker muscles;
Low blood sugar;
Heart problems;
Obesity;
High blood pressure;
Or no visible symptoms.

Types

Here are some of the most common types of metabolic disorders:

Acid-based imbalance - an imbalance in the body's plasma pH.

Metabolic brain diseases

Glycogen storage diseases - the body struggles with storing sugar which then leads to pain in the muscles, being tired all the time and having low blood sugar levels.

Disorders of carbohydrate metabolism - these are a group of disorders related to the breakdown of glycogen and affect the nervous system.

Lysosomal store disorders - that's caused by defected enzymes and there are around 50 inherited metabolic diseases in that category, most of which rare. Gaucher's disease, Tay-Sachs Disease, Mucopolysaccharidosis, to name a few.

Urea formation disorders - that occurs when the urea cycle is interrupted. Then, the body can't remove its toxins and some of the side effects might even be life-threatening.

Peroxisomal disorder - with this condition, a person's enzymes inside cells don't function well. That turns into Zellweger syndrome or Adrenoleukodystrophy.

Causes

First of all, that's genetics. Most of the types of metabolic dysfunctions are inherited and their symptoms can be seen in early childhood. The main reason is usually a missing enzyme or one that is not working well. Such gene mutations may be inherited by many next generations.

Another group of causes is the environmental factors. Lack of physical activity, obesity, a poor diet and bad habits such as smoking all promote metabolic problems.

Other causes or factors that might lead to developing a metabolic disorder include:

Menopause;
Insulin resistance;
Diabetes;
Cardiovascular diseases.

Treatment

The treatment begins by making permanent lifestyle changes so you can reverse the effects of factors that might have caused the occurrence of any symptoms of a metabolic dysfunction. Here's what works best:

1. Eliminate certain foods and drinks.

Some food groups worsen the metabolic dysfunction. So if you're looking to fix your metabolism and live a healthy life again, you should start by eliminating them from your diet.

The consumption of any type of fast food has been proven to cause metabolic problems in people of all ages. That includes **packaged and frozen foods and processed products.** They not only lack the nutrients real foods have but are also filled with additives that cause chemical reactions in the body and interfere with its regular functions.

Examples of such products that are most common in daily life include cheese, cereal, ketchup, margarine, dried fruits, flavored nuts, low-fat yogurt, French fries, white bread, and more.

The next thing you should watch out for is **sweeteners**. They have certain ingredients that even lead to diabetes. Avoid sugary drinks too and things like diet soda, for instance, as they contain artificial sugar as well. While coffee has many health benefits, be careful not to order anything with additives in it which will turn it into an unhealthy food choice and risk factor for developing a metabolic disorder.

Alcohol, when in big doses and too often, is an enemy too. It leads to increased triglyceride levels and high blood pressure, which then affect the metabolism negatively.

2. Lead an active lifestyle.

The next step you should take on the journey to fixing your metabolism is adding exercise to your week and doing it almost daily. No need to get obsessed with working out, though, or to count your calories and wait for weight loss. As we're now discussing how to prevent the symptoms of a metabolic dysfunction, all you need to do is move your body more often.

That means taking walks, jogging, stretching, hitting the gym, or else that you would enjoy. The desired outcome here isn't losing fat, although that will happen naturally, but seeing the other side effects of regular exercise. Such as lowering your blood pressure and cholesterol and reversing insulin resistance.

3. Ditch your unhealthy habits.

Smoking is the first thing that comes to mind in this category. You can't keep doing it if you want to have a well-functioning metabolism and live a long and happy life.

4. Get to your ideal body weight.

Once you take action upon the first 3 tips and don't see progress, you'll need to put in some more effort and actually get rid of the fat on your body. Obesity has side effects that contribute to having some types of metabolic disorders so you need to prevent that and lower the risk.

You already know how your metabolism works and why exercise matters. In the next chapter, you'll find out how to calculate your ideal body weight, after which you'll be given the right foods to eat to get in shape and make your metabolism work faster. All this combined will lead to good health.

5. Turn to a specialist.

When nothing seems to work, you can see a specialist. It's possible that you might need to take a medicine to lower blood pressure, keep your diabetes under control, or else, in order not to increase the chance of a metabolic disease.

Now you know how metabolic dysfunctions occur and what to do and not to do to avoid one or prevent it from progressing. Time to move onto the next chapter of the book and take another step towards your journey to fixing your metabolism.

How To Calculate Your Ideal Body Weight?

Let me start off with what your ideal body weight is and why it's important before you see an easy way to calculate it and begin the metabolism diet.

What is ideal body weight?

IBW is the optimum weight a person should have to be healthy. It depends on a few factors such as height, age, and gender. An average individual who achieves this target will live long.

Calculating that desirable digit is important if you want to be in top shape. It's also the healthiest body mass for a fast metabolism. The ideal body weight is different for men and women. How much you weight depending on your health and body composition is also key as it's the only way to set a specific and healthy goal when on a diet.

Being both underweight and overweight can decrease your life span and lead to plenty of side effects you don't want to experience. With the big number of obese people in the US and across the globe, it's important to take better care of our body. This starts with knowing how much we should weight for our size and age.

How is it determined?

There are a few simple formulas for determining your ideal body weight. Keep in mind you can't have an estimate if you're pregnant or breastfeeding, have a serious illness, are an athlete, or else. This is used for average people with normal or no physical activity who want to know how far they are from the optimum weight.

The most basic equation for your IBW includes age, gender and height. Here's a calculator you can use.

Once you calculate that, you can get an idea of your body mass index too, or BMI. This is another important measure that has a lot to do with the desired weight and is derived from your weight and height. There are more complicated equations and tables you can use, but the standard body mass index formula will work well too. Here it is.

Benefits of achieving and maintaining an optimal body weight

Everyone's talking about losing weight and getting in shape. But few realize the real reasons why that matters. What's more, the ultimate goal here isn't to just burn the fat on your belly or be toned. Many people can lose track of dieting and become underweight, which won't lead to a healthy and happy life either. That's when your IBW becomes the ultimate objective, not just getting to it but maintaining it (which shouldn't be hard once you change your eating habits and start exercising regularly).

Let's see the exact benefits of this:

Lowering the risk of heart diseases. - The right body weight is key to preventing heart problems. Also, it's a solution to recovering faster after a heart disease.

You'll avoid the dangers of having excess weight. - These include arthritis (as there's much more pressure on your joints), high blood pressure, diabetes, high cholesterol, back pain, irregular heartbeat, asthma and sleep apnea. Other health risks include infertility, vitamin D deficiency, eating disorders, anxiety, and depression. Obese people have a higher risk of a stroke and cancer. So as you see, anything that will get you to your ideal body weight will be an advantage and can save you many diseases and health issues down the road.

Feeling lighter and being more active. - Maintaining an optimum body weight means you'll have the energy you need to move as much as you want in daily life. You won't carry around too much or too little weight and so you can freely use your body to train, lift things, do your job, and more.

Improving your sleep life. - Another great benefit is that you'll sleep better. Not only with you avoid sleeping conditions such as apnea but you'll also breathe normally and will get enough hours of solid sleep without waking up. That means the next morning you'll be energized and in a good mood ready to reach your goals in life.

Stronger immune system. - You need that to fight diseases, burn fat and produce energy for your cells so they can restore and renew.

Fertility. - Obesity is closely related to fertility in both men and women as it causes hormonal imbalance and affects the reproductive system. Losing weight and getting to your ideal body weight is one factor that can contribute to improving your fertility.

Happiness. - A person with fewer health issues to worry about will be much happier than those who are underweight or obese. You'll also enjoy life more and do new things as you'll feel lighter and positive.

Increased self-esteem. - Feeling comfortable in your skin due to being in a good shape means you'll be confident in your abilities, won't shy away from new people or avoid social life. That leads to plenty of opportunities, expanding your circle and being in a stable relationship. Many people only find the right partner once they are confident in their bodies and don't have weight problems. That's because they go on dates and are more open. Over time, this is one of the reasons for a healthy sex life too.

Longevity. - As a result of all of the above, your lifespan will increase.

Now you know what IBW means and how it's determined. And most importantly, once you calculate it you have enough reasons to pursue it as a goal as it can turn your whole life around.

Truth is, even the smallest weight loss can help you see most of these benefits. That will help you build momentum and keep going. By opening your eyes for why optimum weight is important to every individual, you won't consider the metabolism diet as something you must do and which is unpleasant, but as an opportunity to get to the desired weight and maintain it for the rest of your life. This will open so many new doors in front of you and you won't allow yourself to lead astray and gain weight again. That's why this chapter of the book is so important - it's a stepping stone to building the foundation of a healthy lifestyle and mindset for the rest of your life.

Metabolism-Boosting Foods

Eating right is the cornerstone of boosting your metabolism. It's all about the foods you consume.

Some slow down your metabolic functions and cause problems in your system, so they shouldn't be part of your menu if you're serious about following the metabolism diet and making a change in your life. Other foods, at the same time, are exactly what your body needs to perform at its peak.

In this chapter of the book, you'll learn more about the things you eat and how you eat them that slow down your metabolism. It's important to work on these first and make some changes to your eating patterns as well as the types of food you consume so you can move onto the next step. Which is a list of metabolism-boosting foods that once added to your diet, will increase your metabolic rate.

Foods and habits that slow down your metabolism

Here are some of the most common mistakes people make in their daily life without realizing that have serious consequences on their metabolism.

Eating less. - People who consume fewer calories than their body needs to function at rest actually slow down their metabolism. The solution here is to eat just enough so you aren't full but also not end up being hungry. Usually, we all know what enough means but our desire to lose weight fast interferes with this. However, if you're determined to reach your ideal body weight and want to fix your metabolism, you need to stop depriving yourself of food.

Not having breakfast. - While there's a diet plan called intermittent fasting which has many benefits on the body and according to which it's okay to skip breakfast and eat during a smaller period of time, when it comes to improving your metabolic rate this isn't the case.

White carbs. - Carbohydrates, or starches, are necessary for us as they are the main source of energy for the body. But there are good and bad carbs. You should stay away from white bread, white rice, white pasta, etc. These are refined grains and contain gluten which can lead to gut inflammation, intestinal problems, fatigue, brain fog and issues with your skin. Avoid processed products and things made of white flour.

Empty calories. - Many people restrict their calorie intake but don't change the quality of their food. They end up consuming empty calories from sugary foods or refined grains. But cereal, cornmeal, cookies, crackers, etc. shouldn't be part of your menu.

Not eating enough protein. - Most people focus on carbs. Sadly, the refined ones. They leave little or no room in their menu for protein and veggies, which is where the real nutrients and fibers are. Protein keeps you fuller and is a great idea for breakfast. It also needs more energy to be absorbed which means you'll burn more calories compared to when you have a meal full of fats and carbs.

Staying dehydrated. - Most people don't drink enough water every day and that keeps the organism dehydrated. Water intake plays a big role in blood circulation, the functions of the immune system and whether or not cells receive enough nutrients. This means that not drinking enough of it will also slow down the metabolism. Experts suggest you should increase your water intake and get to 8 glasses a day. Additionally, drinking it cold makes the metabolism work more to heat it.

Sedentary lifestyle. - Sitting in an office for the whole day is bad for your metabolic rate. While most people simply say they don't have any time to exercise daily, there are many more things they can do. The point is to be moving and to enjoy it, not to be at rest at all times. That means using your car less, having a daily walk, using your free time to be in nature and go jogging or cycling.

Bad grocery shopping habits. - People go grocery shopping without a list and end up buying what they see. It gets worse when they don't take a minute to read the label but assume low-fat means healthy. Most of the products you buy are high in sugar and have artificial trans fats and many additives that cause chemical reactions and hurt your metabolism. Start eating organic products and go to the store prepared with a list in hand.

You eat out. - If you're always in a hurry when grabbing a meal, it's easy to go for the unhealthy alternative. If you meet with friends over a meal and often eat out, then temptations are everywhere and you might often overeat or mix all kinds of food groups. All this leads to being overweight and missing out on ingredients such as vitamin D, iron-rich foods and omega-3 and omega-6 fatty acids. But all these are necessary for a strong immune system and the avoidance of health conditions. The solution is to prepare your food at home and bring it to the office and to avoid eating out most nights of the week. When it does happen, go for the veggies and protein and have as much as you want from it. Be careful with the alcohol too. Social events make you forget about time and you can easily have a few glasses without noticing.

Metabolism-Boosting Foods

Coffee. - Let's start with the beverages. Coffee and green tea are the 2 things you should be drinking aside from water. Anything else is somehow bad for your organism's functions. Caffeine is proven to speed up the metabolism and thus encourage fat burning. It's a stimulant and affects the nervous system which then signals the body to break down fat cells. That's why drinking one or more cups of coffee in the first part of the day is a good idea and you can keep doing this even when you're on the metabolism diet.

Green tea. - One of the many antioxidants in the magical drink that is green tea helps us burn more calories. There's caffeine in it too.

It's now time to the list I promised earlier with all the great foods you can add to your menu that will increase your metabolism naturally.

Broccoli;
Blueberries;
Olive oil;
Almonds;
Coconut oil;
Chilli peppers;
Eggs;
Kiwi;
Carrots;
Salmon;
Tomatoes;
Oysters;
Brown rice;
Garlic;
Lentils;
Lemon;
Curry;
Chia seeds;
Cacao;
Quinoa;
Cabbage;
Oatmeal;
Avocados;
Kale;
Apple side vinegar;
Chicken;
Pumpkin;
Apples;

Tuna;
Cinnamon;
Pears;
Celery;
Walnuts;
Turkey;
Onions;
Grapefruit;
Peanut butter;
Spinach;
Lime;
Papaya;
Organic beef;
Mustard;
Watermelon;
Bananas;
Asparagus;
Ginger;
Eggplant;
Brussels sprout;
Grapes;
Lettuce.

These are the foods you must eat as often as you can so you can transform your metabolism and increase your basal metabolic rate. All the wonderful changes as a result of that will only begin once you make permanent changes in your eating habits.

Conclusion

Congrats on making it this far. Your journey to fixing your metabolism and any health issues you might be having is about to begin. Now you have all the information you need to do it right, without any drastic diets, big lifestyle changes or restrictions.

Your goal is to find the balance and that takes time. Each of the habits and actions mentioned in the book is something you should work on one at a time. Don't be in a hurry. You're doing this transition once and you'll reap the benefits for the rest of your life.

The metabolism isn't just the body's ability to burn fat. It's where life begins and ends and the solution to fixing most of our conditions and problems in the future. You don't need to starve yourself to speed it up. You just need to know how it works and take the necessary steps such as regular physical ability, avoiding the foods that slow down the metabolism and replacing them with those that boost it.

Never forget that everything in your body is energy and chemical processes activate all necessary functions. That energy can flow freely thanks to a fast metabolism as it's what extracts the nutrients from food when digesting it and then turns it into energy that cells and organs use to exist, repair and grow.

There's fuel in food, especially in the items listed in one of the last chapters. But there's no way you can get to them if your digestive system isn't working well. A slow metabolism doesn't burn fat and makes you tired. You lose muscle and gain weight because of that. But with the natural ways to reverse that process that you read about in this book, you'll be ready to fight any dysfunction you might be noticing in your body.

There are a few popular myths about the metabolism that people believe and which make them give up on trying to take control of their health and life span.

The first one is that our metabolism is inherited and we can't slow it down or boost it. That's wrong and you can choose from a list of things on how to change it. That could be by adding physical activity to your daily schedule and doing both anabolic and catabolic exercises. It could be by ditching bad habits such as smoking and drinking. Then, you can improve your sleep, drink caffeine and consume more proteins, which will immediately affect your body weight. Over time, such changes transform your body composition and you become a healthy individual who can move freely, is confident and burns enough calories even at rest.

Another myth is that everyone has the same metabolism. We included all factors the metabolic rate depends on for a reason. Whether you're a man or a woman, the number of stressors in your life, how active you are, how old you are, and many more - all these are what the speed of your metabolism depends on and you can easily use this information to your advantage. When making changes and going on a diet to speed your metabolic rate naturally, you should take these into consideration. Most often women realize they have hormonal imbalance and need to take care of this first, before seeing improvement in their metabolism. Men, on the other hand, form muscles more easily. So with some physical activity, they can create muscle mass and thus use more energy to burn fat.

Make a list of the genetic, lifestyle and environmental factors in your life that have something to do with your metabolism. See which ones slow it down and what you can do about each.

Improving your health means constantly keeping the negative influences in mind and avoiding them as much as possible while filling your days and surrounding yourself with positive factors that contribute to your well-being and are good for your body and mind. That might mean eliminating people in your circle who aren't good for you and keep complaining and judging or forgetting about your favorite snack if it's white carbs or a sugary drink.

These sacrifices are necessary. Basically, you need to unlearn the old way of eating and thinking about your metabolism and adopt these new behaviors we talked about throughout the book. Once you do that, your new norm will be a healthy lifestyle that even reverses the signs of aging and restores damaged cells. You'll feel great about yourself and others will start noticing how you're changing.

Soon your appetite will be under control and you won't crave sugar at any moment of the day. You'll know exactly how it affects your metabolic processes and that it's just not worth it.

Fixing your metabolism isn't just a diet plan. It's an opportunity for a whole new chapter of your life. One where health problems aren't present, you appreciate your body by taking care of it and have the energy to do all you want with your time.

Let your journey to a healthier life and faster metabolism begin no later than today. Sit down and make a few lists. Write down the bad habits you've developed over the years that you need to slowly remove. Then, choose your favorite foods of the list of metabolism-boosting ones that you want to add to your men first. Make sure you calculate your ideal body weight and set this as your main objective.

Good luck!